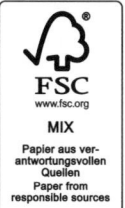

Books on Demand
ISBN 978-384-822-0366
Copyright & Right for Translation
or further Use only by the Author
Dr. Karin Wettig
Munich, Germany, September 2012

Dr. A. S. Karin Wettig

Facelifting without Surgery –
Face Care & Make up for Girls &
Boys between 13 & 103!

Hollywood Secrets for Natural Beauty at any age

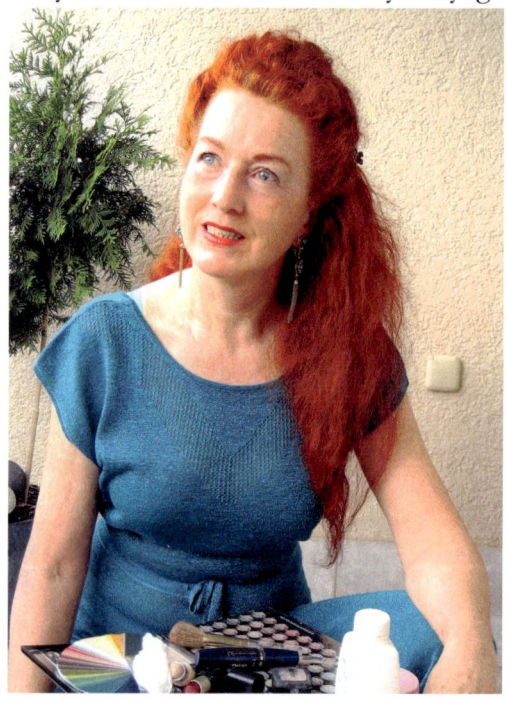

Table of Contents

stir well, put on your Skin, ready...

Look Here this Face celebrates its 60th Birthday!

...

Daily 10 Minutes for Your Neverending Youth Make you Feel Good!

Even if you and I might be no Hollywood Stars or Celebrities, we have one thing in common and that is a face which is aging every day for one day...

The face on the book cover just celebrates its 60th Birthday! Like every human face it shows characteristics of the biographic story of 6 decades. Some crow's feet tell you that the person with this face loves to laugh. A pair of dark circles around the eyes may reveal that the owner is somehow thin-skinned and sensitive and cried some bitter tears over the years. Emotions may have changed like the weather in Germany. A few lip wrinkles don not hide some worries, which left a trace around the tender contour of the lips, a typical sign of elder ladies, in retreatment. Moreover a tendency for dry skin and the lack of pigmentation of the ivory skin of naturally redhaired persons who have to be very cautious with too much sun, increase the danger of early skin aging and early development of wrinkles.

This challenge of my personal type made me look with interest at natural beauty and healthy skin care. Moreover some nutrition allergies and intolerance of bread and yeast, a hypersensitivity against products with a high percentage of histamine, made me dive into the field of healthy nutrition and natural solutions. It was a real challenge to stay beautifully young looking under these conditions for my face when some reddish spots of a skin irritation merged with many small freckles during the period of the hormonal change. If pubertary youngsters suffer from this, I understand that very well and can tell them my story too.

Against all odds and inspite of many little diseases in life the owner of this face feels happy and in wonderful harmony with her younger looking face. How is this possible?

In her youth she would not have won the beauty competition for Snow Whites with her flamboyant curly and thick red hair. She was called often "red Fox" in the streets of her native town. She would not have been a beauty queen too with her strikingly hooked nose she inherited from her father, if not engaged in character rolls like the French Hollywood Star, Gérard Départdieu.

As Colour and Style Analyst she engaged herself early to care not only for her own attractive outfits, but also for a perfect business appearance of her customers and friends. As a musicologist with a passion for opera singing she could experience how make up has to be prepared for intense stage lights and television appearance to overcome the heat and dry climate of studios and concert halls.

Behind the scenery she researched what Hollywoodstars and their body make up artists do for a star presentation and to turn an every day face into a shining star. But this was not enough. Much later she detected by chance during a journey to Egypt and Israel how healing the mud of the Dead Sea is and this discovery made her develop her personal anti-aging beauty care, presented in this book. The formula is unique, easy and made from only three components everybody can find in normal shops. This formula garantuees a perfect basic cover for the face for every day. No further powder, make up or complicated actions needed anymore. It is just ready within 5-10 minutes.

You can mix it easily with the skin care products you might prefer personally and it can be integrated any time into your individual care line. Moreover this mixture of products which are even drinkable as a remedy for the intestine has a healing effect for dry or irritated skin, especially in cases of neurodermitis, which is proven by doctors who tried it out. The combination of these products creates an effect of looking 20 years younger by regular daily use over several months.

Just try it yourself, you will like it. Enjoy the test!

Morning: Your first Gaze in the Mirror…

Without Care – a nude Face like Eve

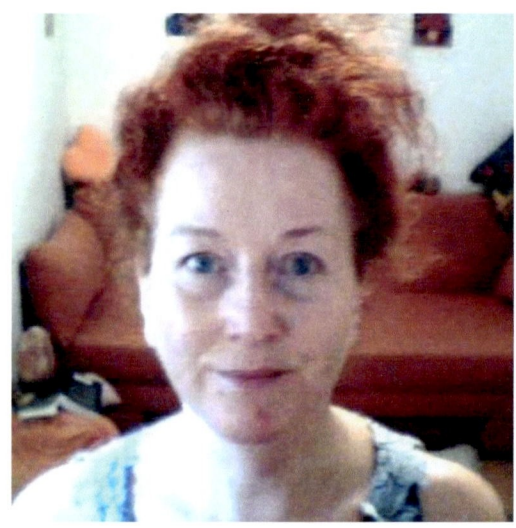

This is what a face of age 60 looks like in the morning, just coming out of the bed; without skin care and even unwashed. A few traces of age, some red spots and typical wrinkles around the mouth and the eyes and sharp contours cannot be hidden in this average face: it shows even some grease after the night although I am a dry skin type in general. In spite of these nude facts, there is a smile just for the photo and no feeling of shame for all these little imperfections. Imagine, normally this face would hide behind the stage curtain and not come up on stage for any presentation or photo before having been cared for thoroughly with my wonder program. Even a partner would find it difficult to have me pose for photos after waking up in the morning: a crazy idea for an idle soul.

Ten Minutes later: a Perfect Result!

Afterwards – only 10 Minutes later

This is what the change looks like after a ten minutes treatment and some light decoration. Some tiny wrinkles of facial expression are still visible: the very fine lines from the alar wings of the nose to the mouth and some fines wrinkles on the forehead. But the facial skin, the throat and the décolleté are covered by a light care, which stays in perfect condition for the rest of the day and might only be powdered lightly in case of extreme heat in the afternoon. Even greasy skin can be treated once in the morning so that no renewal is needed for the day. It is only a question of the percentage of the mixture of the ingredients.

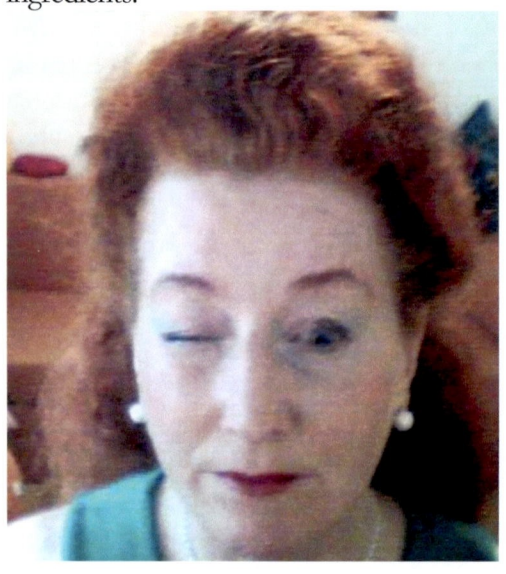

Facial Clarification, Basic Care, a light Styling with some Decoration, in total only 10 Minutes is possible!

The investment into three natural components and 10 minutes of your precious time for this beauty treatment every day is worth while as every person can see on these photos. My example is taken with a simple webcam only and 40 years of practice are a living proof.

What is the secret behind a young face at over 40, 60 and even 80? The treatment is a cocktail from three special components mixed with your personal preferred skin care. I will describe this precisely in the next chapter. In addition there is a cover treatment for uneven or red spots and at the end only some light colour accents to highlight your personal beauty factors – eyes, eyebrows, eyelashes and lips. For men there are also some good tips how to contour a male face without being noticed.

Even without powder this face stays in perfect condition for the day or a great evening appearance if wanted. If somebody is too lazy even to apply this and invest the 10 minures a day, this person might not wonder that at age 50 she or he will need Botox Injections to upholster the wrinkles or even a beauty operation for a facelifting. You can be sure that botox injections or laser treatments and even facelifting operations have no permanent effect over the years. It might come worse, because mistreated sensitive skin feels hurt and reacts with anger and inflammation to this surgery. Remember that even a sunburn is in the memory of your skin over the years.

Cosmetic surgery is very expensive and often not successful, not to mention the pain and the need to repeat them after some years. How much easier it is to apply every day three components with your cream and look with 80 still as if your were 50 or 60.

In my little practice book here I wish to share with you my personal beauty tips and tricks of the last 40 years and motivate you to install this daily self-spoiling manoeuvre in your daily life. Your beautiful face and a good feeling of higher selfesteem will accompany you during your day and give you a protection against the daily stress.

Even if you have to stand up 10 minutes earlier every morning you should enjoy this ritual in front of your mirror and feel the magnetic energy shift you may also get by looking for some minutes intensely into your own eyes. You will feel more energized after this and your great grand children still will talk about their beautiful grandmother or grandfather when you have past your 65th or 70th birthday. Your kind face expression and your glowing skin will be not only a model for your children but also for all other persons around you.

Take your chance tob e a model for your world!

I deeply desire that this little book might be read also by youngsters and adolescents from age 13 on and especially by men. All those who are now at school or university or in the age of the grand children I would like to have, will notice that these tips help also against puberty pimples and are perhaps even better than some spot creams. Practicing them it will be easy to make them a daily routine when after some days a silky feeling appears on your skin. Moreover skin allergies like rosacea, eczema and even psoriasis react to Silicea and salt from the dead sea as is proved by several therapies. But you need not to travel there as I did to find out more about it. You can just buy the readymade powder, mix it with water and apply it yourself. Both, silicea and dead sea mud, have an antibacterial effect. If you still argue you might not be able to invest daily 5 or 10 minutes, you can prepare the mixture of components in a box and put them ready for use in your fridg. If that doesn't help you might control your daily schedule as you seem to be in danger of burnout and other stress illnesses which are the no.1 factor for death in industrial countries and also a cause for many other chronic diseases.

Take these moments for your self and your picture in the mirror: not only your skin will be grateful but your energy field and your better facial presence will be noticed by your surrounding after some days. It is a positive investment in your personal development for the upcoming years of your life if you use your daily skin treatment as a mirror exercise for selfvalue.

Even Morning Grouches do wash - Skin Purification or Clarification – what is best?

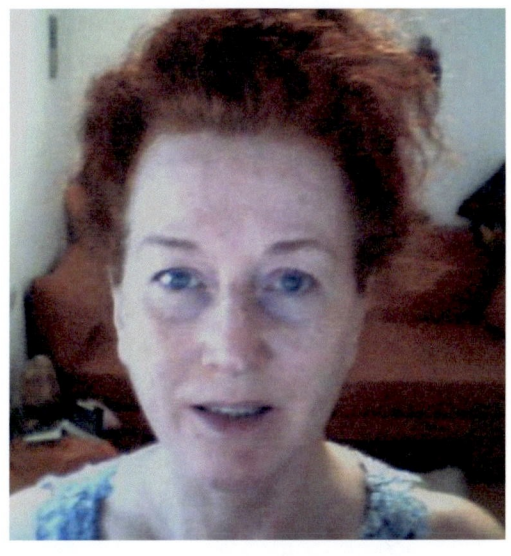

Clarification with Aloe Vera Facial Tonic – if you prefer Water or Soap, you might choose what you like…

The daily clarification of the face should be adapted to the skin type. Greasy skin tolerates products with alcohol to degrease or a good soap. For sensitive skin this would be the end. For dry skin like mine it is absolutely forbidden to use any alcohol on your skin. A mild skin tonic or a distilled water with a calming ingredient like rose bud, camomilla, citronella or lavender or orange flower if you prefer one of them because of the nice perfume, is better. Aloe Vera is the best to give humidity to your skin as this plant grows in deserts and is able to store water for a long time together with a lot of minerals. Be sure that I don't do here advertising for products; I only give you some ideas what is useful. Everybody is allowed to use his or her personal preferred cosmetics.

To talk about water as a skin clarification I have to admit that water is different in any town. As we have here in Munich water with lots of lime, I prefer to use mineral water or cosmetic products without aggressive ingredients for my face. Aloe Vera is my preferred facial tonic. Sometimes I even use a drop of lemon and some yoghurt to calm my skin with a mask before the weekend comes.

Here you can see a picture with the instruments for daily skin clarification:

A bottle with facial tonic, some coton pellets and cotton buds…

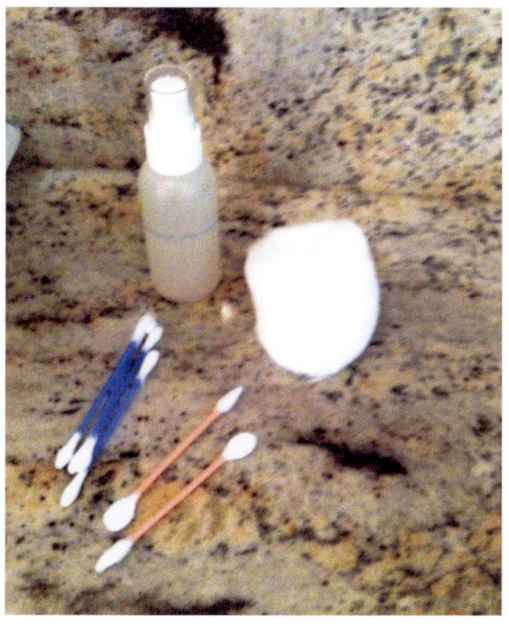

Expert Tip for Skin Clarification besides Facial Tonic with Aloe Vera – Lemon & Yoghurt

For daily use intensively degreasing products are not recommendable in general even for greasy skin as they motivate your skin to produce more grease and destroy the natural bacteria caring for the skin. It is better to change the nutrition or diet slightly. Once per week a deep skin purification is helpful. It can be done with water steam, a visit in the sauna or a skin clarification product with vitamin A acid. Vitamin A acid enters deeply into the skin and cleans it from inside out. A drop of lemon in your facial tonic or even applied to your cream will work wonders against free radicals and Bulgaria yoghurt can not only be applied to the face as a mask but also to the genital area. If you prefer a cleansing milk, just take what you like.

A gynecologue and a skin doctor told me years ago that many women use to much soap for their body care and the genital area. This destroys the natural regulation of the skin. Natural products like yoghurt, milk based treatments or light natural oils are better than anything else. Just try it.

When I see during my visits in our nearby swimming hall how young mothers torture their little babies by using so much shampoo on nearly hairless baby heads which tends to burn in the eyes together with water when it is washed out and causes always a real clamor under the showers, I ask myself often if this soap treatment is really needed. Every kind of soap destroys the acid factor of the skin and causes dryness which makes your skin age earlier. I tend to use water to rinse my long hair often instead of shampoo every time or a facial tonic, just to refresh the scalp. That is completely enough after swimming to feel fresh and clean. If you have a tendency for greasy skin or hair, just use a very mild shampoo then.

Eyes - Care for the Reflectors of your Soul...

Eye Care against Shadows & Wrinkles

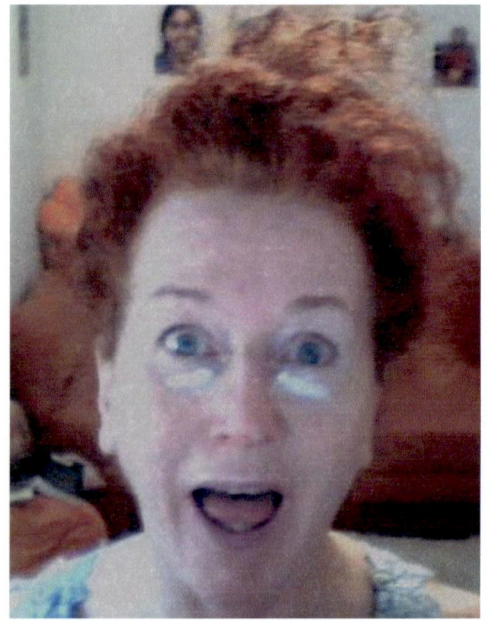

Expert Tip for Eye Care – Baby's – under the diapers cream or a good cold cream

The number of eye care products against crow's feet around the eyes is endless and confusing, because every week you'll find a new product advertised in your droguerie market. They promise reducing even wrinkles but I never found one of them really useful for that purpose. There is caffeine lotions easy to apply around the eyes like a stick which help during the day for tired eyes, but not against wrinkles.

Even pharmacies overflow with special health products for the eyes, where the price seems to guarantee more effect. The effect is mostly to feel in your slimming purse, not so much in your face. To grow old is related to having more wrinkles and a face with more sharply defined contours. It cannot be avoided completely, only set to come very late. When you look around you can see that singers tend to have nice face expression even in their late age. Some actors who live healthy also seem to be more resistant against wrinkles. My experience is that singing and fitness for the face like Benita Cantieni's Faceforming help a lot to avoid early face aging. Many people forget that gymnastics is not only useful to form the body but also to hold nice proportions in your face. Especially the eyes need such a training as they are often overstrained by reading and computer work or inner stress.

With the hormonal change the skin around the eyes tends to become more transparent and that way the veins and the blood circulation gives more shadows around the eyes. My personal tip for the eye care is to use a special cream which is taken for babies under the diapers. This cream is produced in Germany by a special anthroposophic company which should be available also all over the world or a similar product. After cleansing the face I always put two spots of this white cream under the eyes and give my eyes a massage from inside towards the outside until the cream is totally absorbed. The shadows of the eyes are then well covered and this cream which is a protection for babies most sensitive parts helps really to protect the light skin around the eyes from free radicals and against many influences. I even use to repeat this action twice or during the day when I feel I need it. Even if it has no sun protection factor it helps because of the dense cover.

My personal product has no kind of alcohol and is available in small packages so that I can take this cream into my purse with ease. Without that cream and my trio of face care products I never would start any travel. For persons over 40 this face treatment is extremely important if they like to look with 60 still as if they were 40. For teenagers it might be helpful to hide the shadows after a long intense disco night or for managers to cover the signs of stress and burnout. But, if you like to look young in your later age, it is indispensable to eat healthy and sleep enough, otherwise no facial treatment or any quality cream would hide the consequences of any stress or excess.

Patient discipline brings up miracles – is an Arabian Proverb. This is very true in case of body care and cosmetics.

Well cared Men are irresistible - Five Minutes daily for his Success! The Basics...

Adstringent & Nurturing in one Step

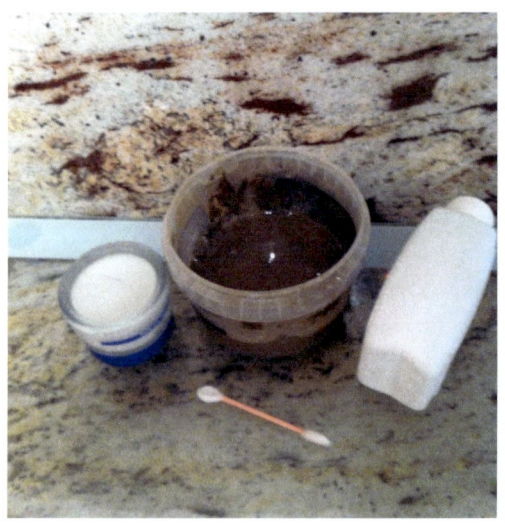

Expert Tip – Silicea & Dead Sea Mud

If men don't like to invest much time for beauty care, I have to admit that I am the same type. I like to be lazy in the morning and a whole make up would just be too much for my morning ritual. Because I love my minutes for the tea and breakfast, I developed my personal recipe rather early in my life. My skin care is a combination of mask, face care, cream and make up in one step. Ingenious - and it really works. I know that every professional aesthetician might exclaim that this is not possible, but it really works. I think only cosmetic and pharmaceutic companies like to make it complicated with a mass of products to make more profit. When they tell you you should use their beauty line it is more or less a good advertising.

It costed me some weeks to try out my personal combination, but now it works not only in my case but for many of my customers. Every person is allowed to use a personal cream he or she prefers as a basic ingredient. I normally like to take a rather thick skin care for dry skin as basic product. But everybody can use what his or her preference is.

First I take a small portion like the tip of a spoon full of silicea gel on my palm and mix it with a tiny portion of natural dead sea mud. The mud is dark brown. Then I combine this fluid with a good portion, normally double of the other products, of my normal skin care cream for the day and mix it like a good cocktail in my palm. This trio of silicea gel, dead sea mud and your personal cream funtions as an adstringent and a nurturing mask and a protection cream at the same time. No need to do a mask, then wait, take it off and put cream on. Just one step and your face is ready for some little decoration with colours.

The photo of my palm shows you the proportions of these three ingredients. The dead sea mud gives the mixture a lightly brown colour which makes it look like a transparent Make up, but your skin type will never be wiped out or covered completely, the result, when it is done in your best way, looks just perfect.

This combination has miraculous effects as the dead continental sea in Israel is not only located several hundred m under the level of normal oceans but is extremely rich in all kinds of minerals because it dried out over more than 6thousand years. It has a degree of bromium which is found in no other salt on the earth and is highly calming for skin diseases. The water carries every person who walks inside and the salt is so intense that everybody has to protect his eyes. As nowadays the face is often exposed to extreme weather changes, climate change and pollution, unnatural fast food and products which make persons addicted, the skin reacts positively to most minerals. The minerals the dead sea mud contains work well against eczema and other skin diseases. I was very happy when I noticed that it works even better in combination with Silicea gel, because crystalline silicic acid as a natural mineral which is encapsulated in earth and stones.

The skin likes this acid very much and it works like a strong adstringent if you take it just by itself on your skin. Then the feeling is that the skin is dried out. For that reason, every body should try out, which portion of silica gel is the best one to be mixed into your face care cocktail. In case the skin is more greasy than dry, you can use more silica gel together with your daycare cream. In case the skin is dry like mine, you would need more humidity and nurturing cream than silica to make you feel good. Silica Gel produces an adstringent cover for your face which stays like a protection for the whole day. This way a person can be sure to have a business day with ease without being forced to look every two hours in the mirror if the make up is still correct or would need more powder.

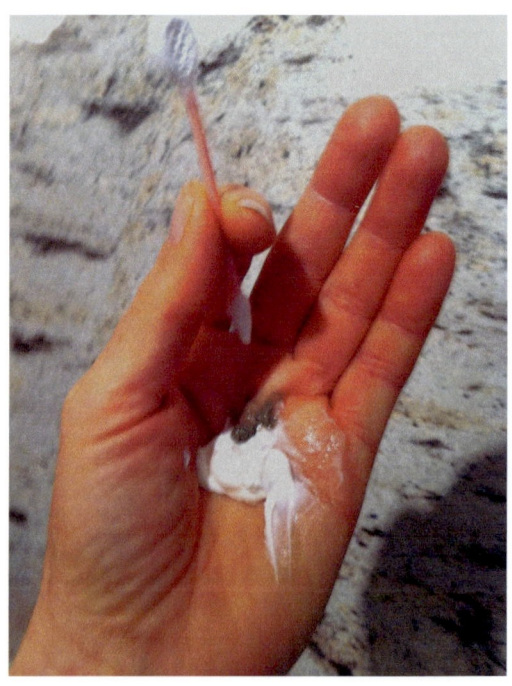

Your day care cream & a small portion of silica gel & only one drop of dead sea mud is just enough.

This little cocktail brings your face to shine and gives you a protecting cover against all influences from outside like wind, weather and pollution. Only when the sunshine is very intense or you live near the equator, you might use a daycare with a sun protection factor as the sea salt can intensify the absorption of light by your skin. This effect is mollified by the dark colour of the mud which looks like a light Make up. The mixture has to be stirred well before you apply it on your face, throat and décolleté and the hands. I use this miracle mixture for all parts of the body where the age is normally noticed first and it saves me time to apply another make up or work with masks to treat my face. I prefer to use the cleansing mask or a nurturing mask once a week during my sauna relaxation after a peeling with salt or almond bran or special wellness products.

I recommended this recipe often to my customers and some ladies reported me that even wrinkles which were existing since several years could be reduced by this method. I noticed from my own trials that I was able to reduce wrinkles on the forehead with my treatment and a combination of gymnastics. It is then much easier too to cover wrinkles and make them disappear completely. Wrinkles around the lips can also be filled with the cold cream or baby cream first and then covered with the special treatment described here.

To work against a face muscle atony you can take the habit to make faces and grimaces during your everyday life whenever you walk to the restroom or have a moment for yourself in front of your computer or at home. Open your eyes wide and imagine to pull your whole face towards your upper backhead. Purse your lips like a sulking kid, lift your eyebrows and roll your eyes around. Look for some seconds with wide open eyes into a light bulb and then rest your eyes until the afterpicture disappears and yawn as much as you can.

Facial gymnastics chases away bad moods and relaxes you deeply. It stops compulsive thinking and helps you to become aware about negative emotions which tend to carve traces into every face. Believe me that a person who uses face gymnastics will be able to smile wrinkle free in her later age.

That's enough tips for now, I think the skin cocktail had enough time to infiltrate into the upper part of the skin and the next step can be taken….

Most Good Things are three – three is Divine: Stir once, that's it!

Make up Basis & Mask in One Step

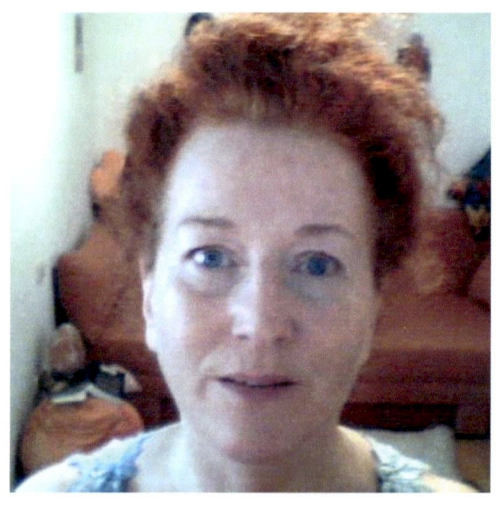

Here the Result of the Basic Treatment can be seen – Adstringent, Nurturing & Cover in one Step.

After you have applied the described miracle cocktail of Silica Gel, Dead Sea Mud and Cream, also over the parts which were already treated with the cold cream or baby cream, your face is well prepared for the application of some decorative cosmetics. If wrinkles or shadows are still to be noticed you might like to use compact make up or a concealer for these places. You can easily choose a product of your taste.

Some Expert Tips for the Choice of a Make up here.

Even if I like to stay without make up in general, I like to give you some tips here for the best choice:

compact make up can be used in dry or humid form. Compact make up has to be applied with a good paint brush of natural animal's hair. Concealer and a cover stick can be used for small impurities and should fit to the colour of your skin.

How to find out this? Now take a look on your palms and check if your skin colour inside of your palms is more blueish, reddish or has a yellow shine. There is a clear difference in the skin colours of various races. The dark haired or black haired type of Southern countries in

Europe and South America often has a blue tendency in his brown skin like Asian people tend to have too. Southern Europian Types like Italians and Spanish people with dark hair often show an olive tone in their skin colour which is also a sign for a blue pigmentation of the skin. The middle European type with brown or blond hair and blue or green eyes can have a yellow tone in his skin which is often extremely clear in redheads with freckles like in Scotland, Ireland or Britain. Even if you don't ask a colour analyst about your colour type which is often defined by colour schemes of the four seasons, you will be able to decide for your self if you are a more redyellow type or a blueyellow skin type. The redyellow skin type is mostly blond, brown or red haired and looks better with warm yellow based colours whereas the dark haired or black haired type has a blue skin tone and looks better with cool or blue based colours. If your skin has a yellow tone, use a make up which has also a yellow undertone. If your skin tends to the blue use a make up with a blue or redblue component. For the choice of Make up or concealer you should know that a lighter colour brings your face to the fore whereas a dark colours cause a face to look smaller. Your make up or eye shadow colours should never be darker than your natural skin tone. If you have a salient nose or chin, you might apply a darker make up on this part whereas eye-shadows should be lightened.

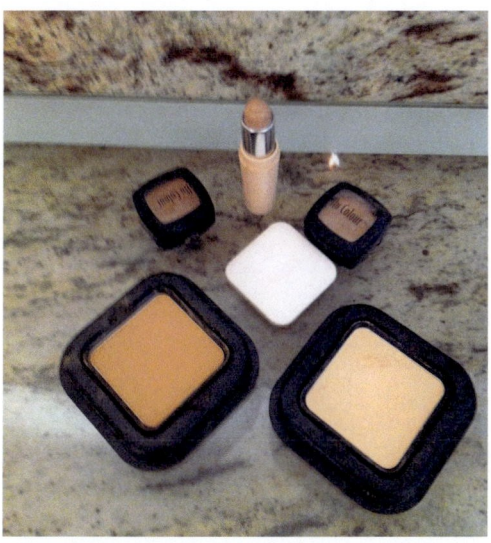

Pimples are treated with a desinfecting product before they are covered with cream or make up. A perfectly prepared teint will look good the whole business day and might only need a tiny bit of powder during extremely hot days. My personal mixture stays normally in good condition for my dry skin even without any powder.

Shine like a Star - Contouring brings Highlights in your Face!

Contours & Colours

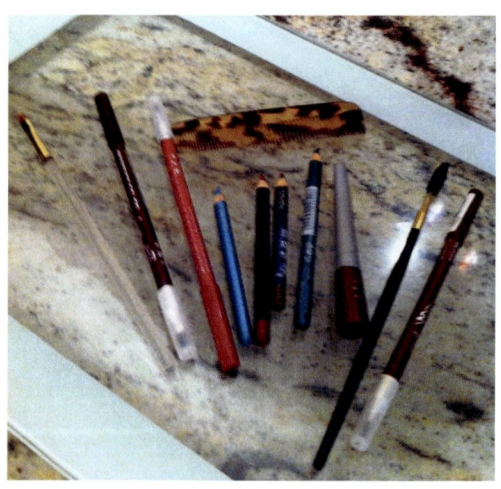

Contouring & Highlighting with Colours helps your Face to Show your Natural Beauty

Now we start with the contouring of the eyes and lips. For my redhaired light skinned type I use copper brown liquid eyeliner which is water resistant as I like to swim. This liquid Kajal can be applicated with the integrated pencil or brush and has to be drawn thoroughly and in a thin line. Don't mark the eye completely like a circle that gives you clown's eyes or a cow – look. Just leave free the inner third and start where the eyelashes start growing. The smaller and finer your eyes, the thinner the contours should be. With a Q tip you can easily take away or correct the line and give it a natural aspect in case you dropped too much liquid on your eye lashes.

Here a good tip for the contouring colours: If you have light eyes don't use too dark colours around them because you take the glow from your eyes away when the eyeliner looks like a dark picture frame around your eyes. Nature knows the laws of harmony and all the colours of your skin, hair and eye type fit together normally. A blond blue eyed type doesn't wear the same colours or make up like a dark skinned black haired type. Black haired persons with dark skin can wear very intense colours. The lip contour is drawn from the inner center towards the outer corner, leave the outer corner free, if you don't like to make your lips appear too broad. Later the lipstick has to be applied over the lip contour. It looks like this, before you go on to the next step:

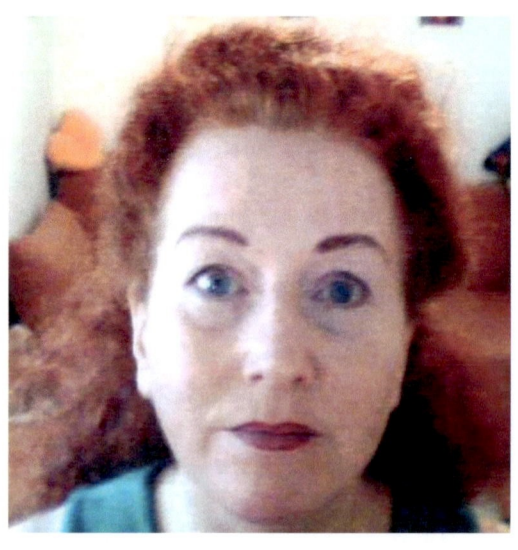

Experttip Contouring – the inner part of the eyes and the outer corners of the lips stay free.

Contouring makes a face more interesting, especially when you have very light colours by nature and a light skin. The nice arch of the eyebrows, kajal and a clear lip form change every body's face into an actor's face when you use these tips correctly: Especially for those who are unaware of their natural physical attractions and how to make them shine, this is a good revelation. The rest is only a tiny step towards a perfect make up and business appearance. There is always a chance to hide characteristics you don't like in your body or type like a too big nose, huge lips or support characteristics you would like to be bigger like small eyes, thin lips etc. For small eyes you apply the contours around the outer corner of the eyes and amplify them with eye shadow. Eyes which are standing far from each other like a contour which comes near to the inner eye corner. The eyebrows have a natural arc where the highest point is at the beginning of the 2. third of the eyebrow. Imagine a line from the side of your nose along the outer corner of the eye and see where the line touches your eyebrow.

Brush away – that's perfect – natural is beautiful!

Mollify Strong Contours

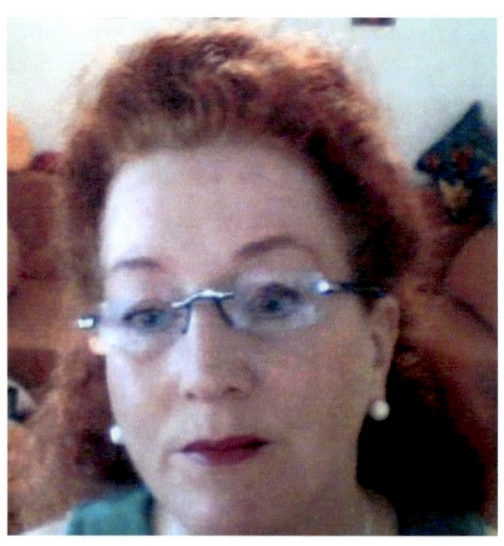

Experttip how to mollify contours – Smooth transitions look more natural.

That is what the contours look like after you wipe them out or break their line with a Q-Tip to make them softer. This face looks more natural even with glasses. I use a small comb to brush the eyebrows which makes me feel energized in the morning. That way the eyebrow colour stays only on the hair not on the skin and looks natural. If you wear glasses check how the contours might look when you wear your glasses. The natural appearance should not be broken.

Lipstick should always be applied over the contours, only very full African lips can wear dark contours, darker than the lipstick which are shining forth. This gives full lips a smaller appearance. If you use lip glow be cautious with it when you have very full lips. For big lips a bit of powder can work well. You would not like in a business meeting that every one stares on your lips…

The right quantitiy of colour in a face needs some sensitivity to be found, but when you have some training for yourself referring to your colour type, it becomes an easy routine. If too much colour went on your face, you can always take away with a Q-Tip or a cotton ball. A well trained colour stylist easily notices if a person chose a useful colour for the type or a dissonant colour.

Well cared Men are irresistible! Five Minutes for his Face make him win!

Face Care in 5 Minutes for Men of any Age without Make up & Powder!

„He came, took a look and won!" was the famous motto of Julius Cesar for his conquests all over the antique world. He won by the first impression the Romans made upon the enemy. He knew that he had to impress to win the battle. He must have done the same with Cleopatra. When my life partner saw how my secret beauty care with the three components made me appear younger while he seemed to age in his face from intense sun and weather influences, he asked me to show him the trick. Easily convinced within three days he complained that the book should also be for men, because they have a right to be beautiful too to please women and to feel attractive to themselves. I felt delighted to see my secrets embellish 100 % of mankind instead of 50% and personally took the photo from his face before and after the treatment. Take a look and judge yourself! As a typical cow boy from the West he used to find creams and lotions unmanly but after the age of 50 he saw that it was useful to change his mind....

I used the same trio mixed from silica gel, dead sea mud and a good anti aging cream and mixed them well. After he had learnt how to cover his sensitive skin around the eyes and the shadows with the cream for sensitive baby buttocks, I showed him how to apply the mixture with a slight massage and allow the face to dry for some minutes. Some greasy parts could be covered with silica gel again or a tiny bit of powder as a concealer for shadows. As men hate powder in most cases, which is my experience from many male customers, I allow them to use only the basic mixture in a way so that there is no grease left over on the face. With some training everybody learns to use just the right portion of silica gel for his skin to be able to stay a whole business day with a fresh face. Here are the before and afterwards photos.

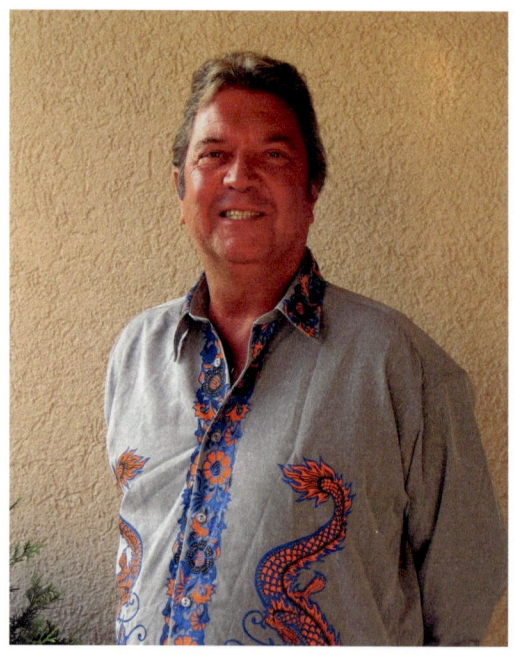

ON the second photo – afterwards – you see that the skin doesn't look greasy and that the eyes look brighter because the eyeshadows are nearly gone. For the hair I simply gave the rest of the mixture on the hair and worked it into the natural curls forming them by combing through with my fingers. A styling for people with no time, but with a good result.

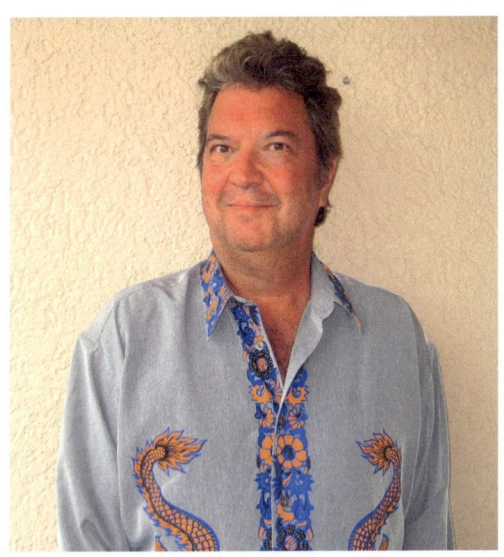

Every man who uses this daily face care will be asked after two weeks if he was on holidays because he looks so relaxed or if he had a new heart flame because his eyes shine so much brighter….

Let them guess!

Make your Type Radiate with Colours!
An Easy Colour Test for Everybody

Blue, Red or Yellow - which Type are you? A Simple Colour Test useful also for People without Experience

To find out what colour type you are, you can work with a simple test by using shawls or pieces of cotton fabrics. Compare some colours under your untreated, uncared natural face and cover coloured hair with a light scarf in a kind of off-white tone. You will notice that every colour has an effect on your face expression. Here you see two colour passports for cool and warm colour types just to notice the difference. The left side has cold colours with more blue and the right side shows warm colours with more yellow as a colour component, because all colours are a combination of the basic colours blue, red and yellow. When you use cotton fabrics it is easier to see the difference, because all shiny fabrics would disturb the impression.

Compare now the colours bright orange with pink under your face in a place where you can have enough daylight. Then compare lemon yellow with bright sunny yellow and Bordeaux read like the wine with a tomato red, then a green with a high yellow component with a bluegreen of the Christmas trees or pines.

IF you wear with pleasure black, white and pink and you get complimented with these colours, you are a cool colour type.

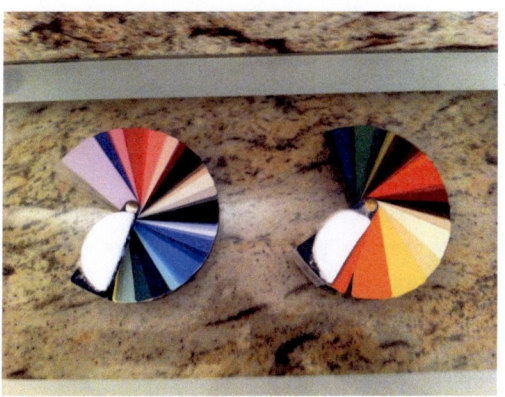

The cool colour type of Southern countries in Europe and South America can have an olive teint which would cause an unprofessional Person to believe that warm colours would fit, but in general it is easy to see that olive has a good deal of blue in it and that the black haired type looks pale by wearing beige or light orange or tomato red.

If you love wearing orange, tomato red, yellow green like in spring and sun yellow, you are a warm colour type for sure and you will find an intense yellow in your skin colour especially when you bronze. Redhaired persons look best in warm colours and you see it that they don't get the dark tan of black haired people, but more a yellow or red tan during the summer months.

Don't feel desperate if you cannot find your precise type as there is a lot of mixtures possible when the parents are two opposite types or you have a mixture in your own appearance like warm hair colour, cool eyecolour and warm skin type. For this reason there are enough colour analysts to check what your authentic preference would be. She can show you which colours make your type glow and which make you look pale or even more fat. As a redhead I know this very well as a white pullover would convince any doctor in my schooltime that I was ill and needed a prescription to stay at home….

When you see blackhaired elder ladies in Southern countries wear beige suits because they think it is decent, they often are shocked when I show them that they make themselves look 10 kg overweight just by using an unfavorable colour. If you have some weight more than you would like to have, be cautious with your colours and use the right make up for your face. Believe me, it makes a huge difference….

I am ready to prove this even to some of the Hollywood stars who think that because of their lives on stage they could wear any colour at any age. When you are over forty any wrong colour makes you look older 10 to 20 years, just try it out, you will notice the difference…

A Breeze of Extravagance in the End...

Set Colour Accents as Highlights — even nearly Invisible ones!

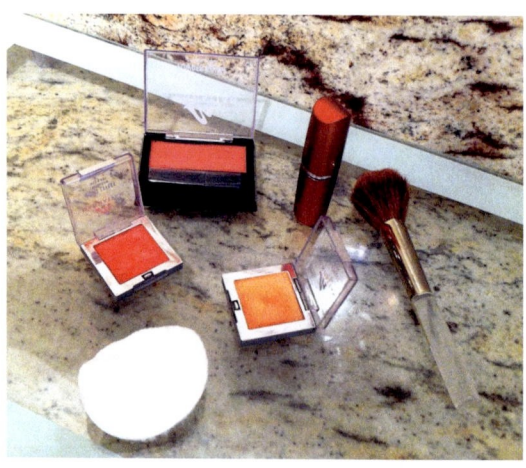

Experttip Make up — Compact Powder for the Colour Type.

Compact powders are very practical for make up as they can be used dry or mixed with water. In dry form they can be applied like a powder over the skin care mentioned here . Just a thick brush of true animals' hair will work well for this purpose. A tiny quantity is enough for the day. The powder should have the same colour type as your skin type so that it is in harmony with your person. There is powders with more yellow or more blue particles. Egyptian red earth is always for a warm skin type and usually not for the typical Egyptian or Southern dark skin type although they seem to love it.

My personal Tipp for powder is not to deviate from your personal skin tan more than three nuances. If you consider your nature you will never apply any extreme. When you use the three components mixtures presented here, you might even renounce on powder in case you found the ideal percentage of the mixture for your skin type.

Colour accents can be set by the application of rouge blush and eye shadow. It makes your eyes and face glow but is not needed in every day life if you don't have time or the passion for it.

I often see young girls with a nude face all tanned with a beige make up. It looks rather naked and unnatural like the face of some Asian dolls. This is only a fashion and will change. Try to find out what colours make you look more lifely and more healthy. For the next photo I used only a little bit of green eyeshadow in the outer corner of the eye and a tiny portion of blush on the cheeks because redheads are often pale by nature.

Be your Personal Hollywood Star every Day! Why not?

Give yourself a Start Signal for your Stage Appearance every Day!

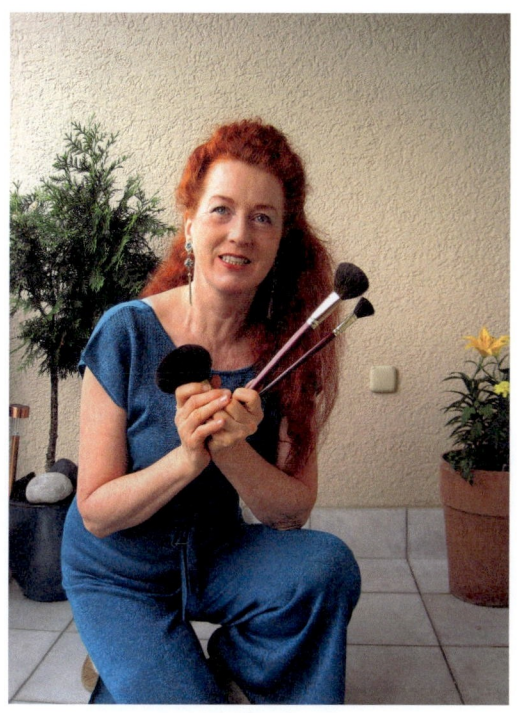

Experttip for Business- or Stage Appearance –
Wear Selfconfidence together with your Beauty!

Many youngsters and also seniors seem to suffer nowadays from a lack of self confidence because nodody seems to notice their hidden talents. They lack opportunities to do what they love and to realize their dreams. Moreover they are told by their parents and teachers to be reasonable, give up their dreams, learn something useful which is wanted by the society or in fashion. My personal way was such an endless hurdling that I understand very well what that is about and how it feels in your deepest heart. Beginning with my father forbidding me to play piano at home seeing me cry for three years because I dreamed about making myself a classical pianist. Later my speaking voice broke and I became fascinated by singing training myself to be a coloratura soprano against all predictions of the singing teachers I ever had.

If you are a pupil, a student, an apprentice or a sales person, a crafts man, a taxi driver or whatever it might be: you have a right to be happy and successful in this world no matter what. Just never allow anybody to kill your dreams or to downgrade you. Every lost battle is a reason to increase one's power. You never know when your chance is at your feet, in this life or the next one. I am sure, it will arrive. Just don't tell your goals to persons who are not believing in your success and don't waste time with false friends like alcohol and druges or games.

Your personal recognition of your own talents and abilities will help you to create what you like. Deeply inside is your hidden potential which comes out of your soul and that can create your reality if you listen to it in silence and meditation.

The person who honours himself and cares about his or her beauty and wellbeing, makes every body's life more beautiful.

Please care about your body, your health, your appearance, your make up, your dress code and your words. Your personality can be seen in the posture of your body, in your gestures, in your behavior and that convinces people if they like you and your company. True self esteem and self love is the best capital you can give to your self and store because it is a wealth nobody can take away from you even in the darkest moments. Even if you believe that you are neglected or not helped by your parents, your social surrounding or your friends you are the only person who can change it. Look at yourself in a mirror and allow yourself to detect this by gazing deeply into your eyes for several minutes without closing your eyelids. This will reinforce your will power and your self respect. Allow yourself to walk through your life with your head held high like a winner. Your body will thank you with better health at any age and you will feel your soul connection.

Self recognition, self awareness brings you near to your soul and to others. Who loves himself, is able to accept the small weaknesses of others with a smiling eye and loves those and himself even deeper for being so human with all errors our race can commit. Love is the best remedy for everything, but many people forget that Christian love includes loving yourself and caring for yourself. When you develop this habit in young years, you will not end in a seniors home being cared for but just take your responsibility and care for yourself every day with fresh intention.

Idols and Models

For young and elder people it is enormously important to have goals and purposes in life. In case you admire somebody for his talents or his expression you have a good reason to emulate him or her. When I gave up on all singing teachers, because they gave me tips without explaining why and what this exercise should bring and my voice didn't become better, I decided to learn from the best singers of the world and I fell in love with late Maria Callas as my best idol. I sat in front of videos for hours and watched DVDs with her opera roles. Even if others smiled about my fascination, I didn't give up and today I can smile because those who criticized me now can hardly believe how I made myself a belcanto voice expert, gave concerts and wrote books about voice training.

Only the person who leaves his routines and walks on new paths, will detect his hidden talents and the courage to master them.

Short Portrait about the Author ...

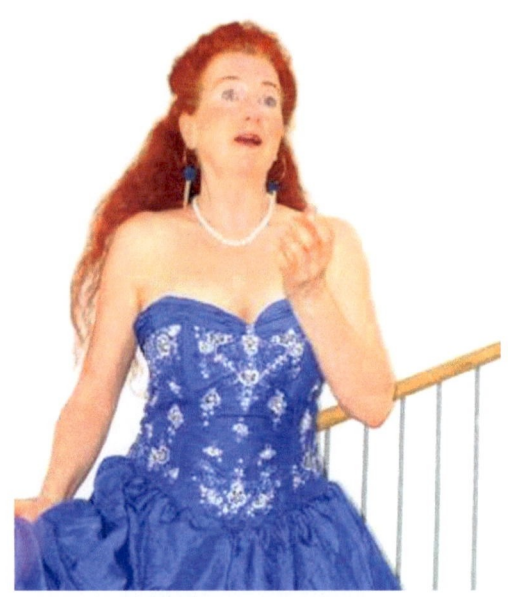

Dr. Karin Wettig, was born in Koeln, Germany, and lives at Munich in Southern Germany. After her translater's diploma, she worked for years as a legal interpreter and translater of legal documents for some German courts at Goettingen, in Nothern Germany. At the same time she studied musicology and wrote her thesis about Carlo Gesualdo da Venosa, a Renaissance composer. She took jobs on fairs, worked in a fashion shop and when the theoretical studies about Renaissance music became too dry she took classes for colour styling and opened her own studio as a colour stylist. After her doctorate her divorce brought a big bang into her life and she ended up with a broken speaking voice.

Karin found no way to make herself a radio speaker as she had intended. Seeking for a solution for her broken voice, she came to Munich took a job and started singing. She detected her passion for opera. Although singing teachers, vocal coaches and voice experts didn't help her much to find the way back to her authentic voice, body training and personal research, breathing exercises and videos of her late model, Maria Callas, helped her finally to repair her broken voice and develop a fine coloratura soprano. Not only sat she for hours at night in spooky churches to train her voice, but researched the literature about Belcanto in various languages.

Her singing adventure journey found a special chapter when she met Ann Reynolds during a masterclass at the castle of Henfenfeld. Her teachings of the Italian Belcanto Method inspired Karin to write her first book – Singer's ABC of Belcanto.

Still not satisfied with the results of her voice, she then gave up on all local teachers to study with the best in the world, Maria Callas and Joan Sutherland by modeling them. A fascinating journey back to the authentic voice of her soul began. She detected her coloratura voice behind emotional patterns of adolescence and traumatic experiences of various lifetimes, researching her inner by hypnosis and selfhypnosis. With her book – Singing like Callas and Caruso – she could finally offer her personal method with body-, breathing - and voice- exercises that had made her broken speaking and singing voice turn into a delightful coloratura soprano.

www.personalitystyling.com

Feedback or Questions are welcome to my email address – <u>Karin.wettig@gmx.de</u>

Love all others like you love yourself, but don't forget to love yourself …